A Book about a Boy WHO BEAT CANCER

Andrew's Story

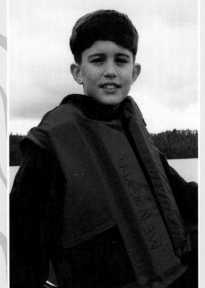

*Text and photographs
by Chris Bridge*

LERNER PUBLICATIONS COMPANY / MINNEAPOLIS

Lerner Publications Company
A division of Lerner Publishing Group
241 First Avenue North
Minneapolis, Minnesota 55401 U.S.A.

Website address: www.lernerbooks.com

Library of Congress Cataloging-in-Publication Data

Bridge, Chris.
    Andrew's story : a book about a boy who beat cancer / Text and photographs by Chris Bridge.
        p.   cm.
Includes bibliographical references.
    ISBN 0-8225-2587-9 (lib. bdg. : alk. paper)
    1. Bridge, Andrew—Health—Juvenile literature.
2. Nephroblastoma—Patients—United States—Biography—Juvenile
literature. [1. Bridge, Andrew. 2. Cancer—Patients. 3. Cancer.
4. Diseases.] I. Title.
RC280.K5 B753   2002
362.1.'9699461—dc21   00-012109

Manufactured in the United States of America
1 2 3 4 5 6–JR– 07 06 05 04 03 02

CONTENTS

Author's Note

My son Andrew had cancer when he was three years old. Six years later, he is a happy, healthy boy who is cancer free, thank God!

During his hospitalization, I looked for books to help him through his experience but was unable to find what he needed. So together, Andrew and I took pictures and notes about what was happening to him. Later, we wrote this story to help him come to terms with having cancer. We hope it will help other children get through it.

When Andrew finished his treatment, I thought we were finally done with this very difficult experience. Instead, as the days unfolded, I realized that Andrew was left with some emotional insecurities. He had a hard time trusting any adults besides his parents and grandparents. When teachers and neighbors tried to relate to him, he was hesitant and uncertain. If someone reached for his hand unexpectedly, he pulled away. The happy, loving boy I saw at home was not the child others were seeing. At first I thought it was a phase he was going through or just his independent nature. But as I put the pieces together, I realized it was something more.

Andrew had experienced many people "violating his space" in the past year. No matter how much he didn't want to be handled, pushed, or poked, his voice wasn't heard. The people we said were helping him seemed to be hurting him. He was confused. He was not in control.

The child life specialist at the clinic where Andrew was treated suggested that I bring him back to the hospital for a tour. He needed to see the oncology floor from a new perspective—as a visitor, not a patient. Being an observer and not a participant would give him a more objective point of view.

When Andrew saw his nurses and doctors caring for other children who were sick, he began to sort out his own experiences. We paged through his photo album from time to time and talked about what he had been through. When he goes for annual checkups, he can look at his doctors and nurses with trust and gratitude. He realizes that these people did help him. They saved his life.

The trust he regained in his doctors spilled over into his relationships with others. Many people can appreciate the Andrew I know.

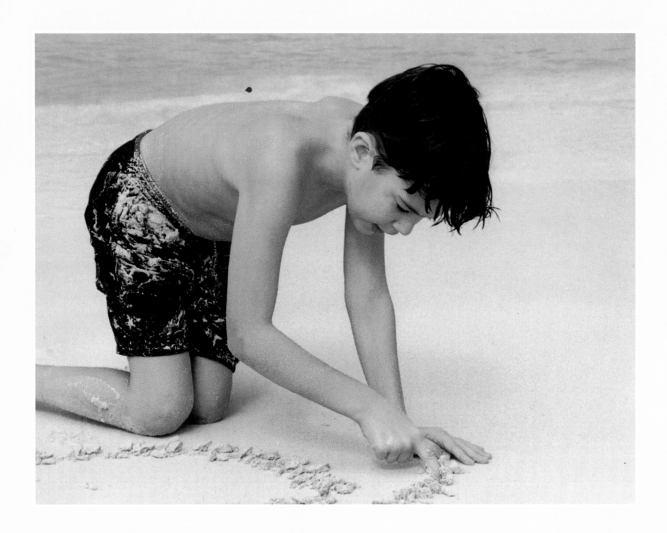

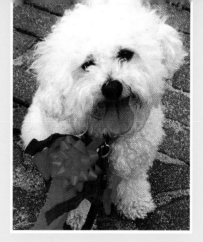

HI! MY NAME IS ANDREW and I'm nine years old. I live in Shoreview, Minnesota, with my mom and dad, my big brother, Tyler, and our dog, Puppet. I like sailing, swimming, math, computers, and playing with my friends.

When I was little, I got cancer and was very sick. But if you could see me now, you would never know it. I'm just like all my friends. I do the same things they do. Most of the time I don't think about when I had cancer.

But sometimes when I'm swimming, someone might notice a scar that goes across my stomach. I tell them it's from my surgery. That's where the doctors took out a lump called cancer. My friends usually just say "Oh," and we keep swimming.

Other times people want to know more about it, and I tell them....

7

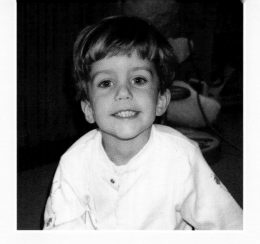

ONE WEEK IN THE SPRING when I was three years old, my neck started to hurt. Then my stomach got very big. When I tried to put on my pants, they were too tight. My overalls still fit me, so my mom helped me put them on. We went to see Dr. Steve.

Dr. Steve checked me very carefully and said he could feel a big lump inside me. He told us to go to the hospital and get some pictures taken so we could find out what the lump was.

My dad came from work to meet us at the hospital. We went to a room with a bed and a machine called an ultrasound. It had a screen that looked like a TV and lots of controls. I put on some pajamas and lay on the bed. Mom and Dad sat right next to me. I could tell that they were worried, but they said everything would be OK.

My mom held my hand while a nurse put some lotion called gel on my stomach. Then the nurse slid a tool, like a little microphone, across my stomach. It felt strange. I pretended the tool was a boat sailing over the ocean. The tool was connected to the ultrasound machine. It made a picture of my stomach by hearing sounds, sort of like the way dolphins search for food underwater. The machine turned the sounds into a picture on the computer screen. The picture didn't look like anything to me. It just looked fuzzy. When the nurse was done, she wiped off the gel and gave me some stickers.

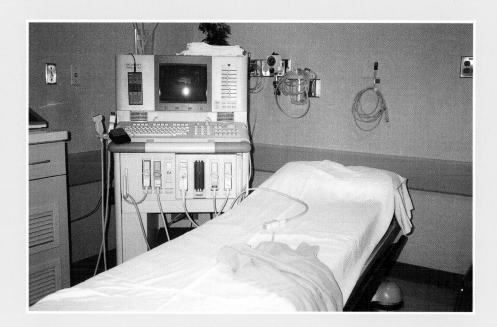

The doctor at the hospital said I should have some more pictures taken with a CAT scan. That's another machine that takes pictures inside your body. A nurse gave me a drink of special juice to make the pictures look more clear. I needed to lie still for the picture, so they gave me a shot that would make me fall asleep.

When I woke up, my mom and dad were talking to Dr. Bostrom. He's a doctor who knows a lot about cancer. He looked at the pictures of my lump and told us it was a kind of cancer called Wilms' tumor. He said I should have it taken out.

The doctor explained things to me so I would know what was happening. A tumor is a growth or lump in the body. Sometimes tumors won't hurt you. Other times they are cancer. The cancer can grow and make you very sick.

At first I didn't really understand what cancer was. But soon I realized that it was different than just having a cold. I was scared. Mom and Dad said the doctors were going to help me get better.

A few days later, we checked in to the hospital. A nurse showed us my room. It had a big bed with buttons that let me move the bed up or down and a television with my own

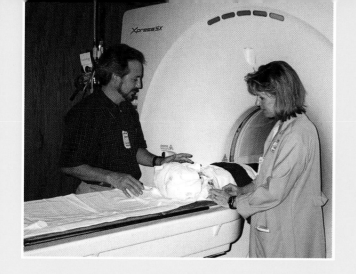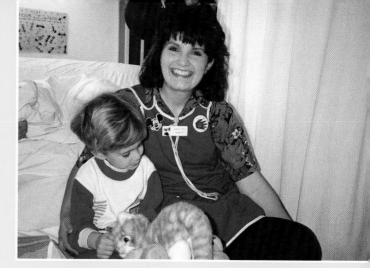

remote control. There was a chair that turned into a bed so my mom could stay with me all night. I brought my favorite books and toys, and we put them on a shelf.

The nurse came in to get a sample of my blood for some tests. She poked my finger with a tiny needle. It hurt for a second. Then she put a Band-Aid on it and gave me some more stickers. After that she brought a tray with juice and crackers and set it right by my bed.

The next day, it was time for the doctors to take out my lump. I had to go to surgery. My mom and dad hugged me before I went into the operating room. They explained what was happening and told me everything would be fine. That made me feel less worried.

During the surgery, I had to be unconscious. When you are unconscious, your eyes are closed and you can't hear or feel anything. A doctor asked me to breathe through a mask that smelled like raspberries. The mask had medicine in it to make me unconscious. Pretty soon it was just like I was asleep. The surgeons cut me open and took out the lump.

When I woke up, my family was sitting by my bed. They were happy to see me, and I was happy to see them! We went back to my hospital room and I rested. The next day, I tried to walk. I felt very wobbly and dizzy. But soon I got stronger and could play with Tyler.

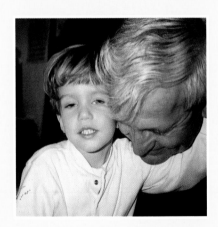

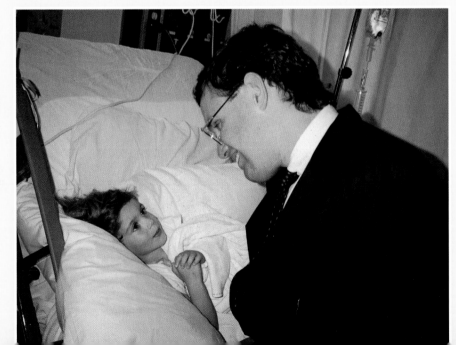

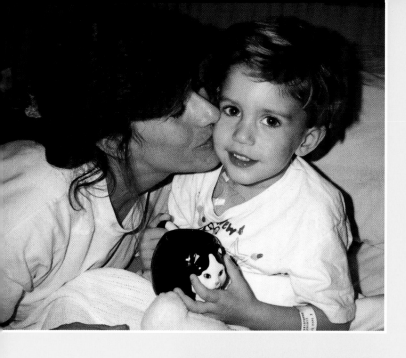

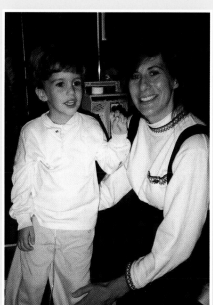

A whole bunch of people came to see me—my brother, aunts, uncles, grandparents, friends, and neighbors. They brought a lot of presents. There were so many balloons, they covered the whole ceiling!

I needed some medicine, but the nurses didn't want to keep poking me. Instead, they put a tube called an IV in my arm. All the medicine went in through the tube and I didn't even feel it. When I was finished taking the medicine, the nurse took the tube and machine away. I felt better every day.

13

I had to stay in the hospital for two weeks. One day I was bored, so my grandma let me play with her camera. I took pictures of her, the doctors and nurses, the Big Bird statue in the hospital, and the fish tank in the clinic. Then Mom started bringing the camera along everywhere we went. We took pictures of everything that was happening to me so I could show my friends and relatives. I wasn't very good at taking pictures back then, but now I have my own camera and am much better at it!

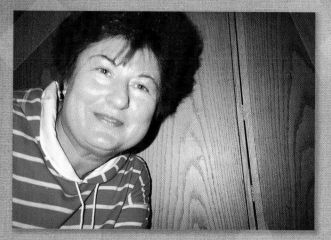
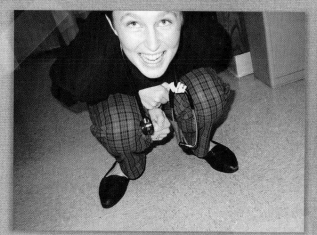
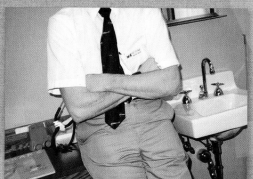
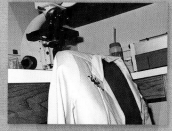
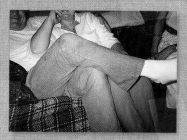
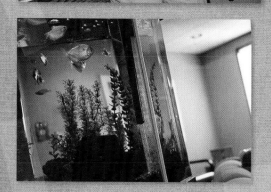
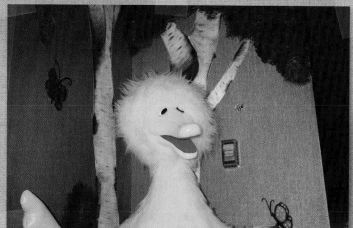

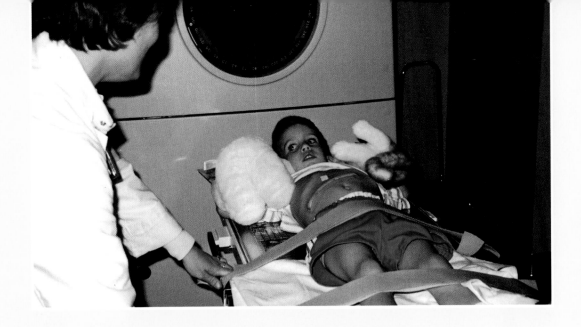

TO MAKE SURE I didn't get another lump, I had to have two
kinds of treatments, radiation and chemotherapy. Radiation
is energy that you can't feel or see, but it can destroy cancer.
I went to the radiology clinic for the treatment. Two nice
helpers, called technicians, took me to a big room with a bed
and a huge machine. I brought two of my stuffed animals
with me. I got on the bed and held my animals. No one
could be in the room with me, but my mom and dad talked
to me and read stories through a speaker. I just stayed very
still and listened to the stories until the radiation was done.
It only lasted a few minutes.

16

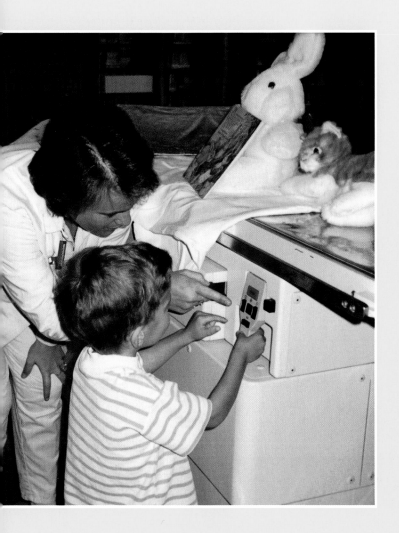

Chemotherapy means taking medicine that fights cancer. I took the medicine through a tube called a portacath. The doctors put the portacath in my chest at the same time they took out the lump.

Chemotherapy was the hardest part for me. The medicine felt cold going into my body. I had to keep taking it every week for a long time—six months. I was mad at the doctors and nurses. They kept smiling and saying they were helping me, but it felt like they were hurting me. I just wanted to be done. I didn't want to go back anymore.

But I did go back. I went because Mom and Dad said the medicine would make me better. Even though I believed them, sometimes I got so mad. Other times I cried. Mom said it was OK to cry.

Then my hair started to fall out because the medicine kept new hair from growing. Everyone gave me hats! I wore them when I went outside, and sometimes I wore them inside, too.

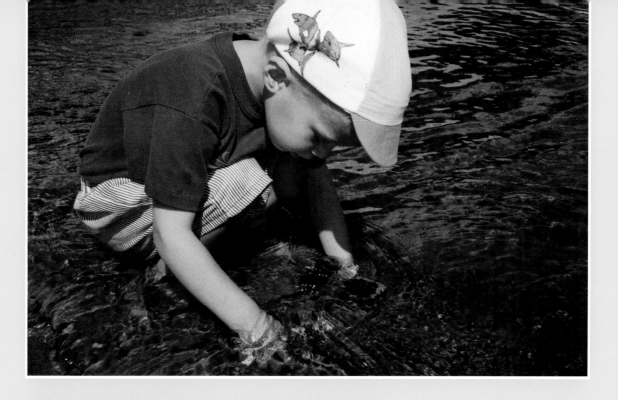

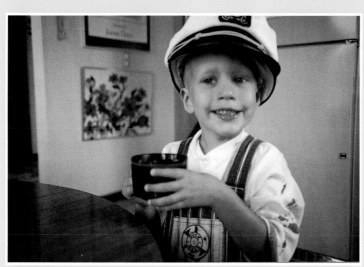

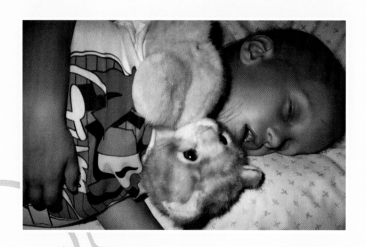

Sometimes when I came
home from the hospital after
my chemo treatments, I felt
tired and I wasn't very hungry.
On those days, I would rest in
my bed, watch TV, and listen
to stories that my mom read.

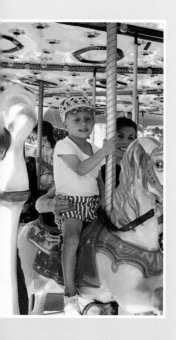

When I felt good, I could do lots of things. I played outside, went for boat rides, and went to the State Fair. I liked riding the carousel there.

I didn't go to preschool in the fall because some of the kids had chicken pox. If I caught chicken pox while I was getting chemotherapy, it would make me very sick. The cancer medicine made my body weak, so it would be hard to fight off the chicken pox. I stayed home, and my friends came over to play at my house. Sometimes I painted or worked on projects, and my mom and I read lots of stories. Tyler and I played every day when he came home from school.

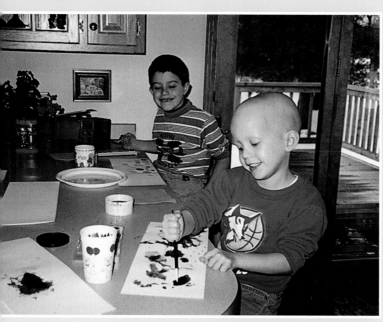

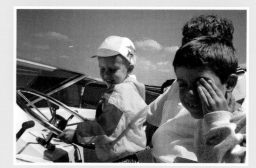

21

I STILL WENT to the hospital a lot. Sometimes it was for radiation and chemotherapy. Sometimes I had to get blood tests to see how healthy my blood was. I also had X rays taken of my chest so the doctors could see how well I was healing and make sure the cancer was all gone. X rays are pictures that show the inside of your body. Doctors have lots of different ways of seeing inside the body!

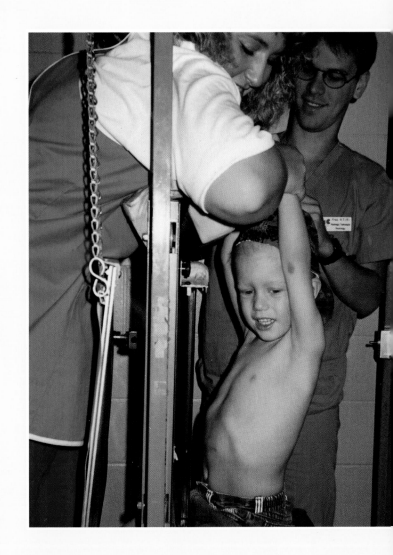

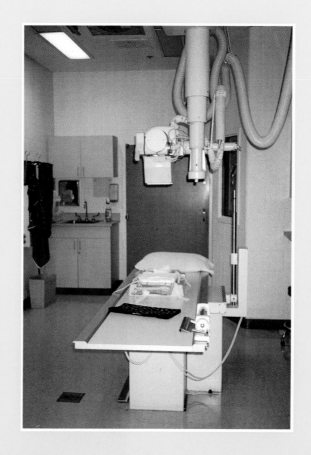

After going to the hospital and clinic so many times, I didn't want to talk to the doctors or nurses or even look at them. I didn't want them to touch me or look at me. I just wanted them to leave me alone.

HALLOWEEN WAS COMING, and I helped my dad carve a pumpkin. I wore a pumpkin costume when we went trick-or-treating, and I got lots of candy. In November, I finally stopped chemotherapy. The doctors took out my portacath. I was so happy! My doctors and nurses gave me a T-shirt that said "Finish Line."

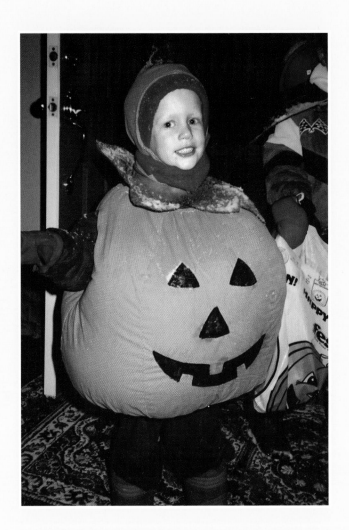

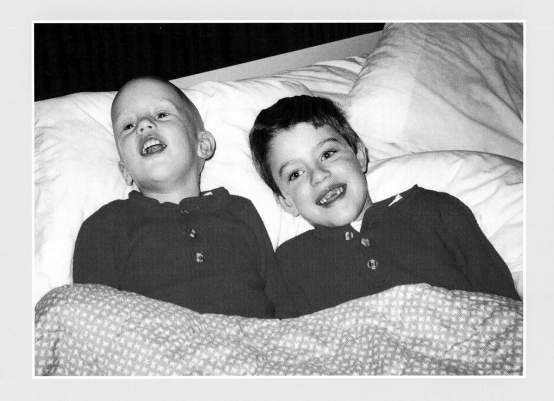

For Christmas, Tyler wanted his two front teeth, and I wanted my hair to come back. Our wishes came true! When my hair first started to grow back, it felt fuzzy. Everyone liked to pat my head.

THE NEW YEAR was like a new beginning for me. I got to go back to preschool. My teacher told the other kids I was coming and that I wouldn't have much hair. Nobody cared about my hair. We all just wanted to play.

By the summer, I looked the same as everyone else. I took piano and swimming lessons and played soccer. I was just like any kid.

I've known three other people who had cancer—my grandpa; my second-grade teacher, Mrs. Nelson; and my neighbor, Julie. They said I inspired them when they were sick because they knew I had cancer and beat it.

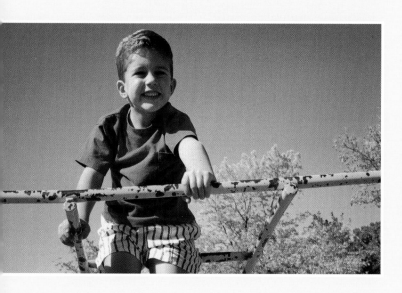
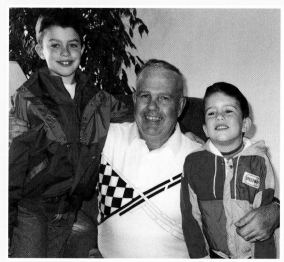

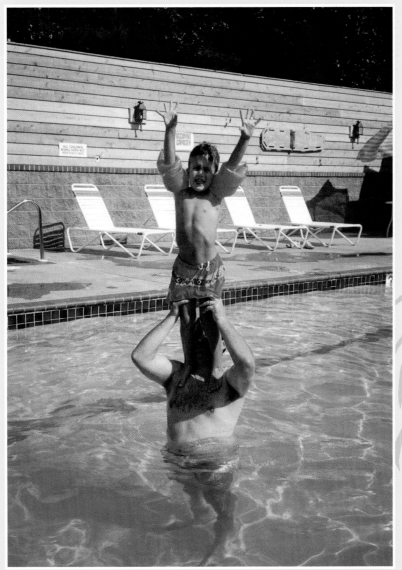

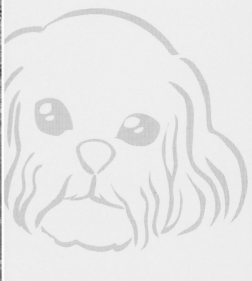

My brother says I inspire him, too. When his teacher told him to write in his journal about someone who inspired him, he wrote about me! I was so surprised. This is what he wrote:

My Inspiration

My inspiration is my little brother. He has gone through cancer, kemo theropy, shots, catscans, ultra sounds, and much more. He inspires me even when he's not there! When ever something bad happens to me I just think about my brother and all he's been through. Then I stop feeling so bad. I remember when he was 3 how he would scream when he got those shots and call names. But he was willing to keep comeing back and getting them. Now he's a normal 8 year old kid. He's only my little brother but he gives me a lot of inspiration.

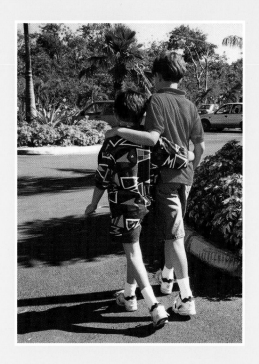

Tyler inspires me, too. He helps me, plays with me, and makes me laugh. He also taught me that, with the help of family and friends, you can get through anything.

These days I only go to the clinic for checkups. When I see the doctors and nurses, I talk to them again. I see them taking care of other kids. I know they are helping them get better—even if the kids don't know it!

Information about **WILMS' TUMOR**

by Bruce Bostrom, M.D.

Andrew was diagnosed with a childhood cancer called Wilms' tumor, a malignant growth arising in one or both kidneys. Typically, it grows to a large size, destroying the kidney before it is detected, usually when a parent notices that the child's abdomen is enlarged or a doctor feels a "mass." The cause of Wilms' tumor is not known, but research suggests that it is due to changes in genes that control kidney growth.

Sixty years ago, most children with Wilms' tumor did not survive, because the cancer commonly recurred in the abdomen or spread to other areas after surgery. Radiation treatment to the area where the tumor was removed decreased the risk of local recurrence, but in many children the cancer still spread to distant areas. In the 1960s, Wilms' was one of the first tumors to respond to chemotherapy treatments. In the 1970s and 1980s, a series of treatment protocols was organized, called the National Wilms' Tumor Studies, to improve the survival chance and minimize the side effects of therapy.

Treatment consists of a combination of surgery to remove the tumor and chemotherapy to prevent the cancer from spreading or recurring. If the tumor has spread outside the kidney or is large, as in Andrew's case, radiation is also used. With this approach, approximately 90 percent of children are cured of Wilms' tumor and can, like Andrew, expect to lead a normal, happy life.

Glossary

cancer—(CAN-sur)—an abnormal growth in the body that can spread and damage healthy body tissue, causing illness or death if not treated

CAT scan—a computer process that takes a picture inside the body; CAT is an abbreviation for *c*omputerized *a*xial *t*omography.

chemotherapy—(KEY-moh-thair-uh-pee)—the use of chemicals or medicines to treat an illness such as cancer

IV—a tube used to give food or medicine through a vein; IV stands for *i*ntra*v*enous, which means within or through the vein.

radiation treatment—(RAY-dee-ay-shun)—the use of energy produced by electricity to destroy cancer cells

radiology—(RAY-dee-ahl-uh-jee)—the use of radiant (light) energy, such as X rays, to diagnose and treat disease

surgeon—(SUR-jun)—a doctor who operates on patients

surgery—(SUR-jur-ee)—an operation to treat illness

tumor—(TOO-mur)—a lump or growth in the body

ultrasound—(UHL-truh-sound)—the use of high-frequency sound to take a picture inside of the body

unconscious—(un-CAHN-shuhs)—unable to think, feel, or sense

Wilms' tumor—a kind of cancer that children can get; the tumor is named after the person who discovered it.

For Further **READING**

For Kids

Carney, Karen L. *What Is Cancer Anyway? Explaining Cancer to Children of All Ages.* New York: Dragonfly Books, 1998.

Clifford, Christine. *Our Family Has Cancer, Too!* Duluth, MN: Pfeifer-Hamilton, 1997.

Cotter, Kelly, and Maury Cotter, eds. *Kids with Courage: Thoughts and Stories about Growing Up with Cancer.* Madison, WI: Wisconsin Clearinghouse for Prevention Resources, 1998.

Gordon, Melanie Apel. *Let's Talk About When Kids Have Cancer.* New York: Rosen Publishing Group, 1999.

Landau, Elaine. *Cancer.* New York: Twenty-First Century Books, 1994.

For Adults

Fromer, Margot Joan. *Surviving Childhood Cancer: A Guide for Families.* Oakland, CA: New Harbinger Books, 1998.

Lazarus, Kenneth, M.D. *Conquering Kids' Cancer: Triumphs and Tragedies of a Cancer Doctor.* Houston, TX: Emerald Ink, 1999.

Steen, R. Grant, and Joseph Mirro, Jr., eds. *Childhood Cancer: A Handbook from St. Jude's Children's Research Hospital with Contributions from St. Jude Clinicians and Scientists.* Cambridge, MA: Perseus, 2000.